THE POWER OF THE SINGLE TALL POLE

CLIMB AND HIKE EASIER, FASTER, FARTHER, AND SAFER

THE POWER OF THE SINGLE TALL POLE

The Complete Guide
to Climbing and
Hiking With
Your
Single Tall Pole

BLAKE CLARK

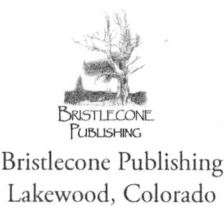

Bristlecone Publishing
Lakewood, Colorado

Copyright © 2026 by Stuart Blake Clark

All rights reserved. No part of this book may be reproduced in any form or by any electronic, mechanical, or other means, including information storage and retrieval systems, without written permission from the author, except in the case of a reviewer, who may quote brief passages embodied in critical articles or in a review.

The information in this book is distributed on an "as is" basis, without warranty. Although every precaution has been taken in the preparation of this work, neither the authors nor the publisher shall have any liability to any person or entity with respect to any loss or damage caused or alleged to be caused directly or indirectly by the information contained in this book.

Written and published in the United States of America

Author: Blake Clark
Cover Photos: David Gebhardt
Interior Photos: Rosemary Burbank
Drawings: Blake Clark

Published by:

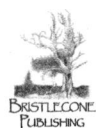

Bristlecone Publishing
Lakewood, Colorado

ISBN: 979-8-218-81895-1
LCCN: 2025921416

ACKNOWLEDGMENTS

I greatly appreciate my wife, Rosemary Burbank, for supporting me in writing this book. She helped extensively with the initial writing, editing and provided all the photographs in the book. Thanks to our good friends, Dave Gebhardt and Dave Rule, for helping with photography on our many hikes, during which all of the photos were taken.

Thanks to my editors, long-time, active, experienced, outdoor enthusiasts Jim and Ann West of Bristlecone Publishing. In addition to editing, they also took the initiative and successfully tested and have now adopted the basic techniques of using a Single Tall Pole. Thanks for your enthusiasm.

A special thanks goes out to Jim DLouhy, Diane Laughlin, and Ken Jacques, three Professional Ski Instructor's Association (PSIA) ski instructors from the Eldora Mountain Nordic Center from whom I took more than 40 cross country skiing clinics during the past 25+ years. They taught me skier evaluation, diagnosing techniques, and teaching techniques, which enabled me to teach backcountry Nordic skiing in the Colorado Mountain Club for 25+ years. I realized their expertise transferred directly to climbing with a single tall pole. Without their skilled training programs, this book would not have been possible. Many thanks.

TABLE OF CONTENTS

Acknowledgments   v

Preface   ix

Introduction   1
  What This Book is About   1
  Definitions   4
    Climber and Hiker   4
    Fall Line   4
    Athletic Stance   4
    Efficiency   5
    Plunge step   6

1. Why a Single Tall Pole?   7

2. The Basics on Using the Single Tall Pole   17

3. Foot Placement and the Single Tall Pole   31

4. The "Plunge Step" Avoidance   49
  Note to Backpackers   57

5. Adapting a Ski Pole   59
  Supplies and Equipment   59
    Pole Preparation   59
    Handle Preparation   59

Epilogue   67

About the Author   69

PREFACE

I learned the importance of the Single Tall Pole from other backpackers on my initial backpack into the Grand Canyon (c.a. 1990). I have since used it on all hikes, backpacks, and peak climbs (including 3rd and 4th class), perfecting a technique I think comes naturally once a person tries it.

My suggestions to others to try the Single Tall Pole are usually met with interesting comments: "I don't understand what you are doing;" "You don't seem to use it very much;" "You must have really good balance;" "I'm fascinated by the way you use it;" "You should write something down."

I have heard comments from strong hikers that, "I tried cross country skiing but I just don't have good balance." I've also overheard excellent skiers claiming their balance is not that good when hiking. Both endeavors require the same basic techniques to stay over your feet. Why the mental disconnect?

I have taught cross-country skiing for more than 25 years. As an instructor, I would not expect giving a few tips on technique to a non-skier to be useful; neither would I expect it to be helpful giving a few random pointers to a hiker or climber regarding the use of Single Tall Pole. I decided it was necessary to write this book to present a process that enables the reader to understand and learn the hidden intricacies that make using a Single Tall Pole an effective and efficient method for climbing and hiking.

The concepts and techniques presented here are not difficult or as foreign as one may first think. Hikers and climbers are already using these in some fashion during their travels. I anticipate the main mental hurdle to learning the new techniques may be to ignore the cultural meme: "If you're going to hike and climb, you need two short hiking poles."

DISCLAIMER—PERSONAL EVALUATION REQUIRED

The decision to use the Single Tall Pole relies solely with you. The techniques employed while using this tool may require serious personal evaluation for both the new and experienced hiker. You may be using two poles because of past injuries, surgeries, balance issues, or physical and medical issues. It is up to you to decide if the efficiencies presented here are compatible with your hiking and climbing goals.

INTRODUCTION

A mind that is stretched to a new idea never returns to its original dimension.

— Oliver Wendell Holmes

WHAT THIS BOOK IS ABOUT

This book explains how you can use a Single Tall Pole (STP) to improve your efficiency climbing and hiking. Its use is very integral for you to maintain effective foot placement, body position, and proper stance while you climb and hike on variable terrain. Its usage is very effective for any terrain that does not require technical climbing gear or ropes. For over 35 years, I have used it successfully while hiking on and off-trails, talus slopes, and boulder fields; on peak climbs (including Colorado's 14,000-foot peaks); and on Grand Canyon backpacks and other canyon hikes. **This may seem counterintuitive, but the rougher the terrain, the more useful your STP is for maneuvering your feet to maintain your stable athletic position through complex climbing situations.**

Many of us are somewhat familiar with the technical aspects of a variety of sports. We understand we're capable of participating in them, and to succeed we must learn and understand the efficiencies involved.

Hiking is an athletic endeavor that warrants evaluation and analysis to search for ways to improve performance. **This is not about competition, but rather about traveling more efficiently for personal health and enjoyment.**

Most likely, many of us started hiking thinking of it as simply walking and not requiring any special skills. Hiking, viewed as an innate activity, was a way to improve our physical conditioning, which, in turn, enabled us to reach backcountry destinations and climb mountains.

The Single Tall Pole system will allow you to use your body more efficiently than the traditional double-pole method. It can be used effectively on difficult terrain where double-pole users may hold them in one hand or stash them on their packs.

Learning to use the STP is not as complicated since many of us are using a basic single-pole technique — without poles — daily in stairways at homes and offices. That is, we use a hand on a railing or bannister while going up and down stairs. The hand becomes a mental reference enabling us to maintain an upright balance point over each foot as we progress. Occasionally gripping the bannister firmly with a little pressure may be all that is needed.

Now, envision traveling on an open-air stairway, without a bannister and the building wall a few feet away from the stairs. Applying the same basic single-hand on a bannister analogy to using an STP, you extend the STP to the support wall, applying enough pressure to maintain an upright body position while keeping your arms next to your body. You are centered over each foot as you walk the stairway. Likewise, on your trails and climbs, the STP provides you with a "bannister" when it is needed.

This book explains why the popular use of double poles, a carryover from snow ski sports (Chapter 1), is not the most efficient way to travel, and why you can hike more efficiently with your STP.

The upper half of the STP has an extended hand grip area. This allows your hands to slide freely and quickly along the pole as needed for you to place the tip of the pole in the most effective spot. Your hands and arms remain near your upper body while using the pole. The additional pole length provides more options for tip placements, frequently allowing you to take multiple strides for one placement.

Improved efficiency reduces muscle, foot and back strain, and joint damage due to impact. The STP encourages you to travel in the upright athletic position (see Definitions on page 4). Its use will enable you to avoid the detrimental effects of the "plunge step" (see Definitions on page 6 and Chapter 4) and possibly extend your personal climbing and hiking career. Your sense of balance may improve as you become accustomed to the strong support the STP provides in maintaining your body's center of gravity over each foot placement (where you put your foot) while you travel over a wide variety of terrain.

I will discuss how you can become more efficient with the athletic stance, foot placement, different stride types, and avoid the plunge step. You will travel more easily as a result of maintaining your athletic stance. The STP is a tool that allows you to freely and quickly adapt to varying terrain features while maintaining this position. You will improve your hiking efficiency by keeping your hands, arms, and torso in a compact unit at all times, directly over each foot, and preventing unnecessary upper body movement.

The information I present is for both novice and experienced climbers and hikers. If you are new to hiking, you may find the detailed foot-placement information useful as you begin using an STP on your backcountry trails. If you are an experienced hiker, you should easily adapt to the single tall pole because of your familiarity with foot placements and the variety of on- and off-trail conditions.

In Chapter 5, I illustrate and describe how you can convert a properly sized cross-country ski pole into a Single Tall Pole.

DEFINITIONS

CLIMBER AND HIKER

These terms are used interchangeably and refer to people traveling or climbing on terrain that does not require ropes or technical climbing equipment. One person's climb may be another person's hike and vice versa.

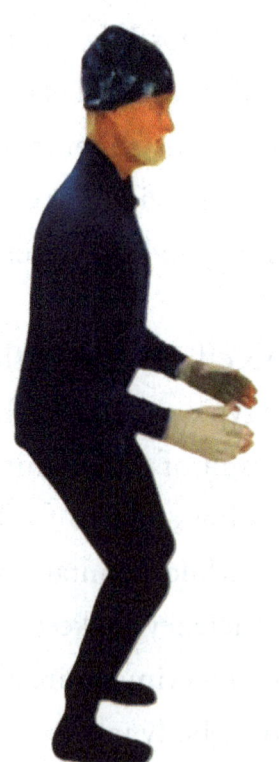

FALL LINE

The fall line refers to the line down a mountain or hill, which is most directly downhill — that is, the direction a ball would roll down the slope without any interference.

ATHLETIC STANCE

The Athletic Stance is the neutral balanced position from which changes of direction occur while keeping the body in motion. Your arms and legs pass through this position on each stride. The relaxed neutral stance is the same for hiking, cross-country skiing and most other sports.

The best way to feel this stance is to stand with equal weight on both feet separated about shoulder width apart, arms relaxed, and shoulders slightly forward. Hop straight up and land on both feet. Note the forward flex at your ankles, the slight bend at your knees, and a slight forward upper torso lean from your hips. This allows for an upward pelvic tilt creating a relatively straight spine. Your upper bodyweight is distributed evenly across the bottom of each foot. As you put your entire body weight on one foot, you can efficiently shift your weight forward to your opposite advancing foot.

The Single Tall Pole is an effective tool for maintaining the efficient athletic position through each stride over variable terrain.

EFFICIENCY

Hiking efficiently allows you to:

1. Transfer and center your body's weight over each lead foot, maximizing friction and therefore stability on the surface underneath, and a smooth stride.

2. Use your larger leg muscles for movement rather than your smaller arm muscles.

3. Eliminate useless repetitive shoulder movement that using double short poles encourages, possibly preventing pain and future injury.

4. Maintain an upward pelvic tilt (tail tuck) to keep a straighter spine, which in turn reduces pressure on your vertebral discs.

5. Ascend centered on your feet and not on your ball joints, and avoid descending using heel strikes, thus reducing strain and impact.
6. Reduce overall stress on your feet, knees, hips and back because your body core remains in a more relaxed upright athletic position.
7. Enjoy more comfort during and after long hikes because there is less impact on your body.
8. Spend less time crossing rugged terrain because your progress is initiated from your comfortable stable athletic position.
9. Extend your traveling range beyond what you originally thought was your limit.
10. Possibly enjoy a longer hiking/climbing "career" because there is significantly less damage occurring to your body over time.

PLUNGE STEP

A descending step, of an inch or two or more, that a climber or hiker makes by allowing his or her full bodyweight to drop, i.e., free fall, onto the lead foot.

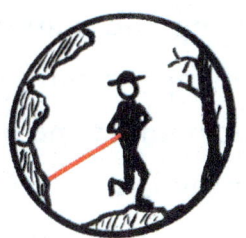

1
WHY A SINGLE TALL POLE?

Nothing is so firmly believed as that which we least know.
— Michel de Montaigne

The successful use of the STP requires you, as a hiker, to think of the pole as a tool, not as an aid. The tool can be used in many different hiking and climbing situations. It does not need to penetrate the ground, as pressure on the rubber tip is all that is required. You use the pole only when needed. Otherwise, you carry it in the neutral position (Chapter 2) allowing for quick responses.

When using the STP, you will be actively evaluating foot placement, body stance, terrain and route of travel, both on and off trail. Hiking with your STP is significantly different from hiking without a pole or with two poles. You will adapt quickly to its easy use as you experience efficiencies in your climbing and hiking techniques.

When we started hiking and running, it seemed to come naturally. When we are young, we can easily compensate for any mistakes. As we age, we often find we need to make changes to how we hike due to aches, pain, and injuries. At first glance, grabbing a ski pole or two seems like a reasonable option, but it's not necessarily the most efficient one.

The alpine ski equipment industry has jumped in to help by providing optional slip-on rubber tips to easily convert ski poles to hiking poles. Few, if any, other significant modifications were made. Hikers used them, at about the same lengths, as though they were skiing. Wrist straps allowed hikers to firmly grip pre-formed single position handles designed to drive a sharp point into hard packed snow.

The indiscriminate selection of a piece of ski equipment as the tool of choice for hikers and climbers overlooks significant differences between relatively smooth skiing terrain and the extremely varied terrain hikers need to deal with. As a hiker, you need a tool that is dedicated to your needs undertaking the extremely variable terrain that a skier may easily glide across in the winter.

The terrain underfoot of a skier is constant in relation to his body. When hiking, however, you travel on extremely varied terrain, requiring your feet to constantly change positions in relation to your upper body. Your feet may be moving up, down, and side to side. They align at different angles to each other as your body inherently changes on each stride while negotiating terrain variations directly under each foot placement. You need to have maximum friction contact under each new foot position, AND you need a dedicated tool for climbing and hiking that enables you to constantly maintain your "athletic position" over your feet. The Single Tall Pole is your tool.

The skier uses two alpine poles to help push himself through lift lines, across intermittent flat terrain, and for turn initiation. The poles are used minimally for actual skiing. The main purpose of the straps is to keep the poles with the skier during a fall. The snow is basically a constant distance from the skier's feet to his elbows. This approximates the proper ski pole length for the skier.

Unlike skiing terrain, climbing and hiking terrain may require you to use your pole at a different length on each stride. You need to use a pole that's designed to be of these varying lengths, which will in turn allow you to adopt new techniques to improve your climbing and hiking efficiency. As an example, one solid STP tip placement, may suffice for multiple double pole placements.

The STP expands the terrain available for tip placement — you can place it farther away from your body than you can a short pole, thus taking advantage of the STP's extra length to keep your body weight over your feet and maintain a proper relaxed posture while crossing varied terrain. The limited range of short pole tip placements can continually shift your body weight away from over your feet and throw you off balance. Furthermore, because the length of the pole necessary for the terrain is always changing, and may be different on each stride (Chapter 2), you don't have to constantly change the length of your pole as you would have to with short poles.

Some claim using double poles can add momentum or speed to their pace. Cross-country skiers can add momentum with a pole plant because they operate on a slippery surface. But in hiking, you do not need a push from behind to help advance your trailing (back) foot on each stride. Using arm strength will force your upper body to lean forward while your feet remain fixed, thus moving your center of gravity forward of your balanced position.

Some feel double pole usage strengthens their arms. Building arm strength is a separate endeavor which detracts from your hiking goals — stability, speed, distance, and injury prevention. Your STP helps you advance these goals by enabling you to hike more efficiently maintaining your athletic posture.

Others extoll the use of short double poles for exercise and health benefits. One reported study indicates walking with these poles can increase the amounts of oxygen and calories you use by more than 20 percent.

But do you really want to expend more energy on your extended hikes, backpacks, or mountain climbs? These are not workouts. They are adventures to be enjoyed!

While skiing and hiking terrains are significantly different, it is important for you to think about the classic cross-country skiing technique — even if you are **NOT** a skier. The basic principles are applicable to your hiking and climbing endeavors.

For example, **what enables a skier to remain upright on a slippery surface while wearing slippery devices on his feet?** The answer — the skier maintains the proper athletic posture with proper foot placements at all times. **And it is not because they have two**

poles. We teach beginning cross-country skiers to ski without poles before introducing proper poling technique.

The classic cross-country skier does not advance by poling. His forward momentum is created by a combination of a forward lean with his hips and a quick downward leg extension from his compressed ankle and knee (the athletic position). This extension forces the grip pattern on the bottom of his ski to momentarily grip the snow and allow him to advance the trailing ski. Repeatedly combining the ski's grip on the snow with his leg extension, he forces his hips forward with each ski lead change, resulting in forward momentum and speed.

The important point here is that the skier must have his entire bodyweight directly over his ski's gripping section on each and every stride. This correlates with the moves you make hiking to advance or change direction with each of your strides. **Like a skier, your hiking efficiency depends on the stability provided when your body core is centered over each lead foot as your trailing foot advances.**

Ski pole plants with arm follow-throughs help a skier to rhythmically maintain stride transitions, just as arm swings do in walking and running. The skier's poling action does add some forward glide momentum over the lead foot, but that glide occurs because of the interaction between the slick surfaces of skis and snow. Hikers are usually not looking for glide!

You can easily incorporate this knowledge of the classic cross country ski technique into your climbing and hiking foot placements. **Using the STP eliminates your urge to use a pole for propulsion and refocuses your technique toward stabilizing your body**

directly over each foot contact with the terrain. (Chapter 2, Flying Buttress).

So why are short double poles considered the ideal tool for hiking? On snow, they stabilize a stationary alpine skier on a slippery surface preparing for a ski descent. This may be the main mental carryover that double poles have for hikers traveling in rocky terrain. But the friction terrain on which summer hikers tread does not have this perpetual slippery threat.

When ascending or descending with a short pole on each side, you naturally tend to orient your shoulders more in line with the fall line. This encourages ascending on the balls of your feet, or descending using your heels as anchor supports — both very inefficient, and possibly injurious, ways of ascending and descending.

When descending precarious steps, you may bend at the waist, extend both arms and poles forward to support your upper body. This significantly reduces the pressure needed for traction on your feet. You are also using your lower back and arm muscles in lieu of the large leg muscles for proper traction. You are more susceptible to falling anytime your weight is not fully centered over each foot placement.

Conversely, using your STP while descending steep terrain enables you to keep an upright body (athletic position) directly over your feet, increasing the pressure needed for good traction, making you less susceptible to falling, and reducing stress on the rest of your body from bending forward.

On steeper off-trail terrain, raising your uphill short pole can shift your center of gravity to the downhill side (danger side). Using the short pole on the downhill side also shifts your weight toward the danger side. In these situations, hikers using double poles may carry both poles in one hand and extend an arm to the uphill side. This upper body motion creates an inverted pendulum effect, making it difficult for you to keep your center of gravity over your feet.

Adjustable double poles do allow for using one pole longer than the other when hiking across steep slopes, i.e., "side-hilling." But the inconvenience of making multiple pole length changes during a hike limits this to special circumstances. As a result, you, like many others, may make do using your preferred pole settings.

When climbing steeper rocky terrain, you may stash your two poles on your pack because they are no longer useful, with the presumption that "poles are for hiking, not climbing." But the STP is a much better tool for climbing rugged rocky terrain (3rd & 4th class), as it allows you to ascend and descend efficiently in the athletic position. From this position, multiple strides may be made with one tip placement through rugged terrain. Furthermore, using your STP enables you to focus more on your foot placement techniques (Chapter 3).

I am offering a new tool for those wanting to improve their stability and efficiency while hiking. Two short poles do give you information regarding left and right upper body tilt, allowing each arm to correct the body core back to a centered position over the feet, which does provide some sense of security.

However, this security is a bit of an illusion. For example, picture a few cross-country skiers clustered and getting ready to start skiing, with hands through the pole straps. Suddenly there is a yelp and a "swish – thud." A skier has instantly fallen either face down or on his back. He obviously lost track of his balance point over his feet, probably fiddling with his gear at the last minute.

A similar scenario can occur with hikers and backpackers using poles with their hands through the straps. Suddenly they can lose traction under their feet, slip and fall. Both skier and hiker were between their poles, but that provided no security against falling. Both are vulnerable to shoulder injuries if a pole impedes the fall, because their hands were trapped in their straps. Obviously, it is more dangerous for you to fall while climbing or hiking than while skiing on a smoother, softer surface. The skier knows exactly what caused the fall. But not always the hiker. I've heard hikers make comments like, "My balance isn't good," or "My shoe soles are too worn, they're three or so years old — I need new boots." (Although each time I could see their boot soles, there was plenty of tread.)

Mother Nature's gravity does not favor new shoes! Both new and well-worn boots require the same proper body position to maximize and maintain friction contact with the terrain. The illusion that hiking with double poles is more secure gives one a false sense that foot placement concerns are secondary to double pole placements. **Hiking with the STP enables you to focus on your foot placements and use your STP as a TOOL to do so.**

Your strategic STP tip placement affords you the stability to keep your body in the athletic position, your weight centered over each foot placement, thus maximizing your friction contact with the terrain. This book will explain how your STP is actually anchored with both hands and arms near your torso, maintaining a stable, effective, athletic position throughout multiple maneuvers.

The following chapters will focus on explaining how you use your STP to improve your efficiency (see Definitions on page 5) by concentrating on maintaining proper foot placements.

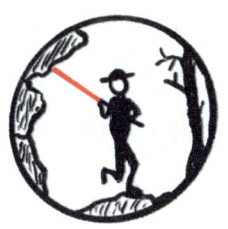

2

THE BASICS ON USING THE SINGLE TALL POLE

One of the greatest pains to human nature is the pain of a new idea.
— Walter Bagehot

Your proper pole length is proportional to your height. It will stand at a height between your mouth and forehead — about 90 percent of your height. You can easily convert a tall cross-country ski pole to make your STP (Chapter 5). Your finished product will have a continuous padded grip zone, from the bottom of the fixed ski handle, covering approximately 40-50 percent of your pole's length. The extended handle section allows you to make quick smooth hand adjustments along the STP, to quickly create your best effective pole length needed, at any given moment. You will replace the sharp ski pole tip with a blunt rubber cane tip, giving you strong support without penetration, allowing you to quickly change pole tip placements.

Your hand is NEVER inserted into the wrist strap when actively using the STP while hiking. Your hands will be continually changing positions along the pole as the terrain continually dictates the different pole lengths needed. There are two uses for the pole wrist strap when you are hiking. It acts as a hand stop when the pole quickly slips through your loose hand grip to obtain a full-length position (Chapter 4, Plunge Step Avoidance), and your pole can hang from your wrist if you need to make climbing maneuvers requiring the use of your hands.

You might ask, "Why keep passing a single pole from hand to hand, side to side, when I can just use two poles?" **The STP does not actually change sides**. It remains in front of you when in use, laterally/horizontally, across the general direction of your travel, regardless on which side the tip placement is required. The following simple process explains how quickly your STP tip can be moved to your left, then right and back again, for consecutive tip placements as you are hiking.

1. Grasp and hold your pole vertically in front of you with both hands comfortably apart (about one foot) near its center. The strap handle should be up and the tip down.

2. Release one hand (either one) and your other hand's wrist quickly rotates the tip to the desired side (either side) for placement.

3. Both hands now adjust and grasp your pole for tip placement. With each change, your hands alternate functions. (Hand functions are explained below.)

4. Loosening your grip then allows you to quickly slip the pole to the desired tip placement point.

You need to make a strategic visual tip placement to ensure the pole angle will be relatively **perpendicular to your support point** on the terrain. You do not randomly poke with your pole in search of support points while you are simultaneously looking for footing. For comparison, note that when you are using your hands for climbing, you will look at the rocks before placing your hand as you extend your arm to a support position — and it's not just because you don't want to disturb a snoozing rattlesnake!

Your visual pole placement is strategic because **you do not want this tip placement to shift** when a single position may be used for several strides. The blunt rubber cane tip keeps your STP from penetrating surfaces, as with a hand, permitting it to be moved quickly to the next spot. The blunt tip only needs to support sufficient **pressure** to keep your body in the stable athletic position over your full-foot print — again using the analogy of the arm and hand extended to the stairway bannister. Because you are not suspending body weight on the pole, the tip pressure via your arms detects whether or not your STP tip placement is stable before you advance the trailing foot. You know immediately before progressing if any adjustment needs to be made.

The strategic placement of the pole tip involves using the STP laterally across your body (**Figure 2-1**, on the next page), then using your **guide hand** and your **pressure hand**. The distance to the pole tip support position will determine where the hands are placed along the pole. Your **guide hand** aligns the STP with your desired tip placement support location, with relaxed fingers, as if you were lining up a pool cue for a shot in a billiard game. You do not need to grip the pole firmly. Your **pressure hand** then engages the pole tip to that point, and your hands and arms anchor the pole near your body's torso to maintain your body's center of gravity over each lead foot during your stride transitions.

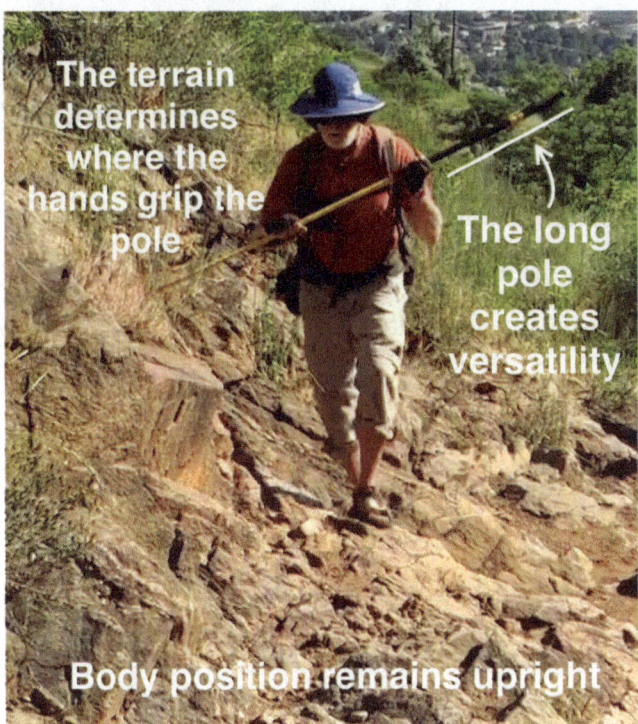

Fig. 2-1

The most useful support points for your STP tip are those closer to right angles from your body, about chest high. A tip placed near your foot makes it difficult for the pressure hand to support the body over that foot because the pressure is going down toward the ground rather than laterally to a support point. As you increasingly change the tip placement laterally to different points away from you, notice how much easier it is for your pressure hand to stabilize your body directly over your lead foot. Your eyes will become accustomed to scanning more horizontally for support points, rather than looking at the area near your feet.

When your STP is not needed, slide your guide hand to its midshaft balance point and casually carry it across your fingers with the strap handle forward. This is your **neutral carrying position**. (**Figure 2-2**) You can readily raise your guide hand's arm and quickly rotate your pole tip left or right if needed for another tip placement.

The STP is only used when needed to support you over foot placements. The neutral carrying position keeps your arms and shoulders relatively inactive when traveling over easy terrain. Hikers using double poles tend to maintain repetitive useless arm motions of planting pole tips on each stride. If you have experienced shoulder dislocation or shoulder pain, you will appreciate eliminating this repetitive motion.

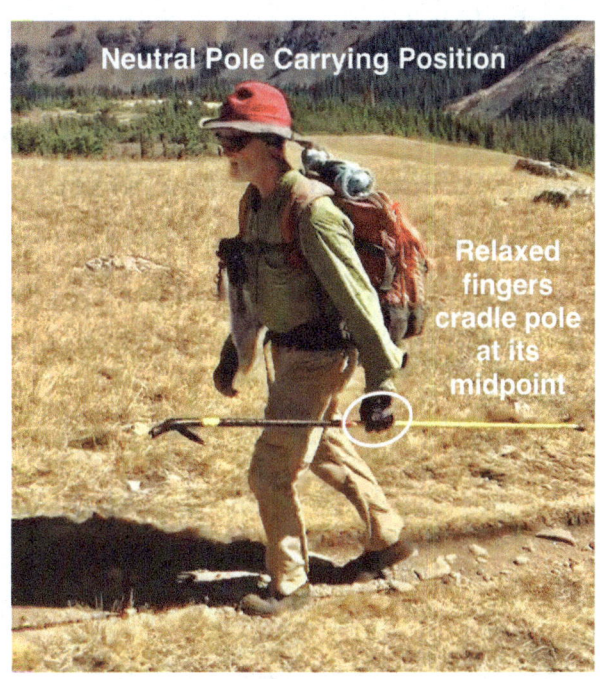

Fig. 2-2

Typically, your STP tip placements are on the uphill side of your body for quicker responses and more support point options. When you need a tip placement, let's say, to your right side, your right carrying hand (now your guide hand) quickly rotates the STP across your body allowing your left hand to become your pressure hand. Your pole is now relatively perpendicular to your direction of travel.

Here is a significant point. When you place the tip of the pole on one side, your opposite side hand will apply the pressure across your body to keep you centered over your lead foot. This may seem counterintuitive that your pressure hand's action is toward the opposite side of your body. **But this allows both of your arms to remain unextended and close to your body, with the pressure toward the uphill side. Your body position remains constant, unaffected by extending your arms laterally, which would be the case using two poles and would change your center of gravity over your feet.**

Visually draw a circle over your body core, including the chest and shoulders from the waist up to your chin. Using the STP, your hands and arms operate within this range as the terrain dictates, irrespective of whether you are ascending or descending. (**Figure 2-3**) This allows you to establish a hiking rhythm while maintaining your upright athletic position across a wide variety of terrain. Your hands quickly reverse roles as either can quickly rotate your STP's tip to your desired tip placement. (Notice, it is natural for the

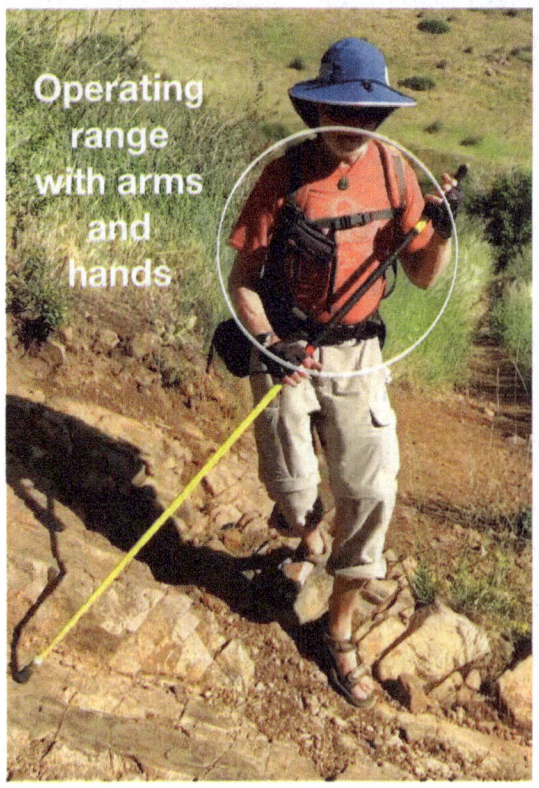

Fig. 2-3

palm of your guide hand to face downward and the palm of your pressure hand to face upward.) When the pole is no longer needed, you may release the grip of your pressure hand and allow the pole to slide to your guide hand's neutral carrying position.

Even if your STP tip placement point may be within your arm's reach, you use the pole rather than a hand and arm. Your body may be only a foot or two away from your desired tip placement location, but you still use your STP. Reaching to use your hand will interfere with your hiking rhythm and body position and delay your next pole tip placement, because reaching with your guide hand to the support point automatically causes your pressure hand to hold your STP out of position on the downhill side of your body.

If you have had experience using double poles, you may (probably will) have a tendency to firmly grip your STP with both hands because your muscle memory kicks in. You may feel it necessary to grip strongly with both hands, even if you haven't been a user of double poles. Either way, mentally you over react because you think "I need support — big-time support!" **In reality, your first need is a strong "support point" at the far end of your STP. Then, you only apply sufficient "pressure hand force" to maintain your body's position over your lead foot.**

Your pressure hand keeps your STP tip engaged as you continue to move away from its placement point, assuming it is still a valid support point. Gripping with your guide hand is counterproductive, UNLESS you need to relocate your STP's tip to another location — that is, a point you select visually and direct your guide hand to target as the new tip location. Your old muscle memory may kick in causing both hands to grip the pole and cause your upper torso muscles to apply pressure to your STP tip placement. As a result, your upper body is no longer centered over your feet, reducing valuable traction and delaying the timing to your next tip placement. Smooth teamwork between your relaxed hands as they operate across your STP enables you to achieve multiple steps or strides with one tip placement.

Now it's time to develop your new muscle memory, i.e., "finesse memory," in your fingers and hands. You may practice this process while hiking. Use your relaxed guide hand to place the STP tip on a support point, then use your pressure hand to place force on that point. Now extend three or four fingertips of your guide hand to the sky, leaving your thumb underneath your STP as you stride forward. (**Figure 2-4**) Feel your relaxed guide hand and the force of your pressure hand stabilizing your body directly over your lead foot. Repeat this process with each new tip placement to build your confidence operating with relaxed hands and arms. Note, your pressure hand can also operate in a relaxed manner when applying pressure. Many times you may only need the strength

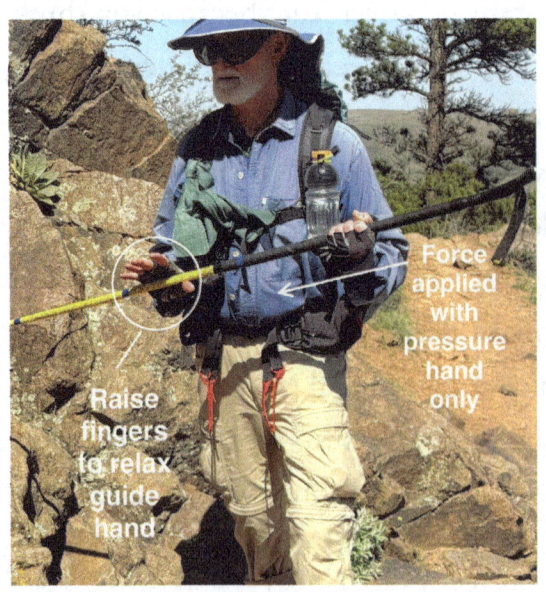

Fig. 2-4

in your thumb and forefingers to maintain pressure. A solid grip by your pressure hand may only be needed briefly for a second or two, as it needs to also continually reposition along the STP handle. This reduces unnecessary muscular activity, making your climbing and hiking more efficient. You are saving your strength and reducing stress. (You are training for your personal "Everest climb" — right?)

Visualize the STP as your personal mobile "flying buttress" type of support. Many medieval buildings and cathedrals have used them to stabilize huge walls, which have lasted centuries. The buttress extends out laterally to a large support structure situated away from the walls of the building. This structure does not need to support the entire weight of the wall. It provides enough pressure (support) to keep the wall in its vertical position.

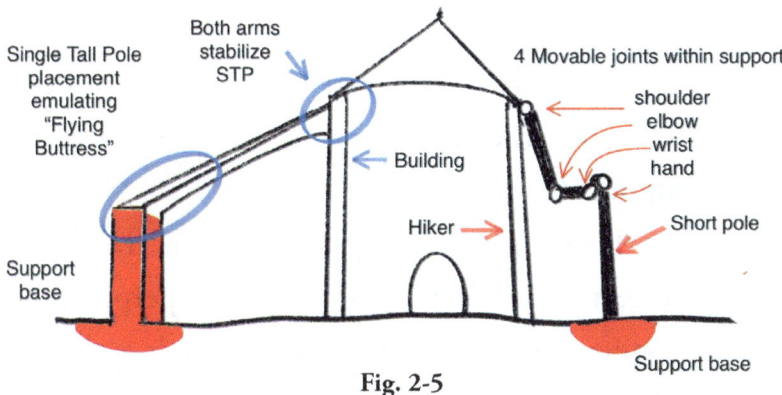

Fig. 2-5

Your athletic stature is comparable with these huge walls. (**Figure 2-5**) The builders did not want them to fall over, and you don't want to fall over either. You are, however, very mobile and therefore need to maintain your "large wall" stature over a wide variety of terrain, adjusting while extending your personal mobile flying buttress — your STP — to rocks, trees, logs or other hillside support points along your route. (**Figure 2-6**)

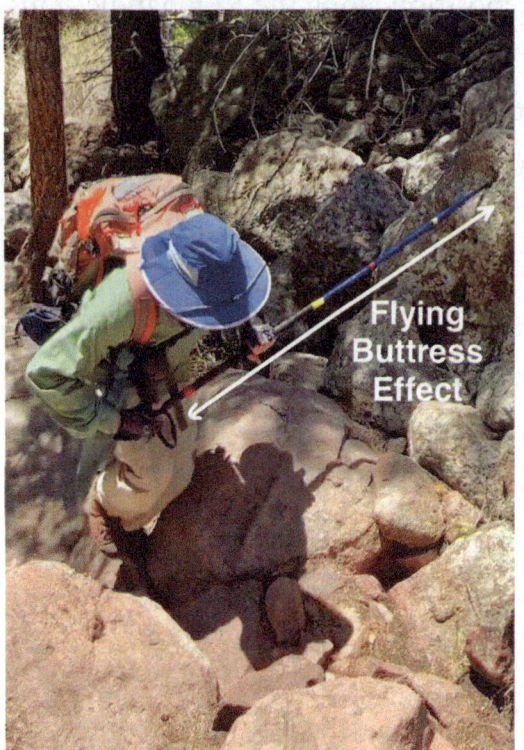

Fig. 2-6

When you properly hold the STP, it is solidly anchored at your torso. This forms a solid straight line support between your torso and a support base. Short hiking poles do not provide this solid straight line of support. They allow needless fluctuations in the body position because these support lines contain four movable joints — shoulder, elbow, wrist, and hand palm — all of which use your smaller muscles to manage support between your body and its support bases.

You may try this simple test to experience the flying buttress stability. Stand near a wall, with your shoulders perpendicular to it, so that with your fully extended arm you can place the palm of your hand on the wall. Set your feet about a shoulder width apart with a slight forward flex in the ankles and knees. Now move both feet about a shoe width further away from the wall so you feel your arm and hand pressure supporting your body's force against the wall.

Raise the foot closest to the wall and notice two important feelings: 1) you have solid body support with the wall (the support base) and, 2) your single shoe on the floor has a **solid friction contact with the floor**. Hold this position while flexing your body and swinging the free leg back and forth, and experience how stable you feel. The STP allows you to bring this experience of stability with you on all your hikes and climbs.

Let's evaluate a scenario (**Figure 2-7**) with a hiker climbing a gentle grade traversing a steep hillside with the high side on his right. He is carrying his pole in the right hand neutral position as he is approaching a rough, rocky section. Then his right guide hand rotates his STP horizontally to align its tip for an uphill side placement as his left hand grips the pole and applies pressure to engage the tip placement. Stepping onto the first rock, he is

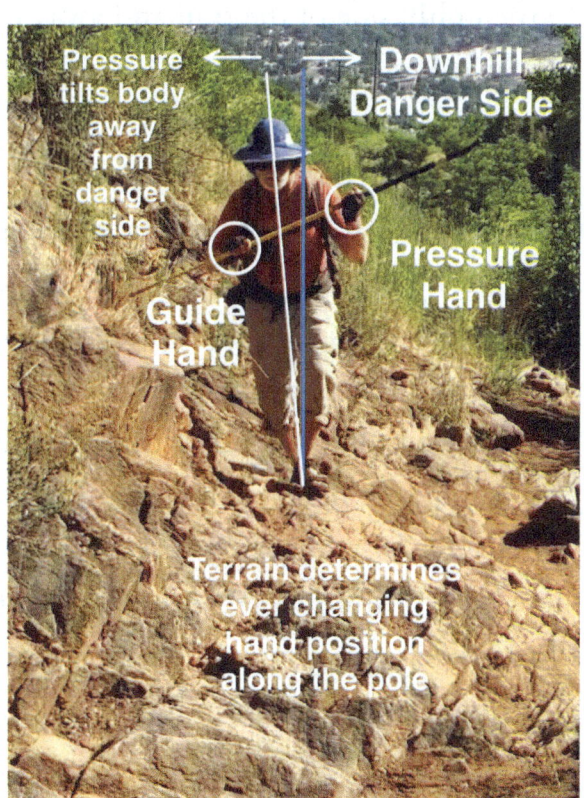

Fig. 2-7

momentarily centered and stabilized on the lead foot as the trailing foot begins to advance.

Now suspend our hiker in time, with his STP tip in place, body supported on one foot mid-stride, and address three important aspects.

First, his STP is solidly anchored across the body torso with both arms and hands near the body.

Second, his STP is providing stability for his body to remain over the lead foot, allowing more time, if necessary, to evaluate the next foot placement.

Third, you cannot see it, but there is a **psychological advantage you will experience** by applying pressure across the body to the uphill side of the trail and away from the downhill side — which I refer to as the danger side. This is mentally reassuring when you are crossing steep slopes.

As we reactivate our hiker, he advances the trailing foot to the lead position and, if necessary, changes the pole tip location. Strategically placing the tip a little farther forward allows him to move several steps with one pole tip placement. His hands change positions along the pole as he moves closer to the tip support point.

It will become second nature to you to rotate your STP to your uphill side hand as the terrain changes, whether you ascend or descend, switchbacking direction across a slope. You will use these basic techniques regardless of the steepness of terrain. With a little experience, you will operate with relaxed hands along the STP, quickly moving its tip to effective placements all along your route as needed.

Your upright athletic position will make it easier for you to scan the terrain ahead and be more effective at determining when and where to make your tip placements. Many times you may see immediate ruggedness ahead and place your STP tip in anticipation of precarious footing, but then realize after placing it, you do not actually need to apply significant pressure on it because your position is stable. But your STP is ready just in case.

This chapter focused on the lateral (across your body) STP technique while keeping both arms relaxed and close to your body. You will use the lateral pole techniques extensively, climbing and descending on your routes, as you become accustomed to effectively anchoring your body with your "mobile flying buttress" over each of your foot placements.

It is important for you to remember the STP is a tool which allows you to concentrate on feeling the stability of having solid foot placements throughout your strides while maintaining your efficient upright athletic position. Chapter 3 will give you more detail regarding how some bad foot placements can be overcome using your STP. These basic techniques will be useful on your descents and transfer to a single arm pole technique for preventing the "plunge step" (Chapter 4).

3

FOOT PLACEMENT AND THE SINGLE TALL POLE

Be sure you put your feet in the right place, then stand firm.
— Abraham Lincoln

The term "foot placement" refers to the point on the bottom of your foot that supports your body directly above it, maximizing the friction between the foot and the ground, making the sole of your boot grip the ground most securely.

The terms "forefoot" and "midfoot" are used in walking and running literature. I prefer to use forefoot because I think it better fits the description. I define the forefoot as that part of your foot in front of your arch, which includes the ball of your foot and your toes.

When in your athletic position, your trailing foot, leg, and hip advance together, with your forefoot already positioned directly under your body. Your forefoot initially engages the ground first.

Then in a split second, your foot and leg muscles engage to support lowering your full body weight onto your entire foot print available with minimal impact to your body. Your spine remains relatively straight as your pelvis tilts bottom forward (as in a tail tuck), because the flex in your forward ankle and knee keeps your body slightly lower (your athletic position). This reduces excess pressure on your vertebral discs. The body's center of gravity over the entire foot maximizes the amount of the sole of your boot in contact with the ground, which in turn maximizes the friction between them (the grip of your boot), thus reducing the chance of slipping.

This also explains why the cross-country skier is stable using slick skis on a slick snow surface (Chapter 1). It is also why your elderly grandmother takes short steps as you assist her across a snow-packed parking lot. She's an experienced athlete keeping her center of gravity directly over each foot on each stride. (Be sure to compliment her on her athleticism!)

Your forefoot placements allow you to avoid the use of heel strikes. Our modern culture has largely adapted the heel strike method of walking, which can be detrimental to your body. When your extended leg and heel hits the ground, a shock force travels back through the knee and hip. Furthermore, your pelvis tends to tilt top forward when using a heel strike, causing more curvature in the lower spine, impacting the vertebral discs, which over time can induce back pain. Additionally, the heel strike makes you more vulnerable to slipping (discussed later in this chapter).

The STP challenges you to continually experience and use the dynamic between your engaged STP tip and your stable body centered over your lead foot placement. With practice, your

experience will readily become second nature to the way you travel. There are two pressure points: 1) Pressure on your pole tip, only sufficient enough to keep you over your full foot placement and, 2) Maximum pressure of your body directly over your full lead foot placement to maximize traction. Instead of putting pressure on the tip, the STP is used as a light support to maximize the pressure on your feet and increase your traction, stability, healthy body posture, and the use of your large leg muscles. **It is the essence of climbing and hiking with your STP.**

Wearing flexible footwear will enhance this pressure dynamic. You can test this flexibility by holding a shoe at the heel with one hand, and the forefoot portion with the other. You should be able to twist your two hands in opposite directions without exerting a lot of strength. If they do not twist, the shoe doesn't pass the flexible footwear test.

Flexible soles quickly transfer more information to you regarding what is directly underfoot, allowing your ankle and leg muscles to freely adjust, maximizing contact with the ground or rock surface as you are ascending or descending steeper terrain. That said, **you should not rely on footwear to solve the traction problem.** Once again, shoes with new or well-worn soles require you to use the same important foot placement techniques needed to enable you to hike and climb efficiently.

It is very difficult for a casual observer to visualize the pressure and dynamic you experience using your STP. The observer may only see an erect person walking over rock-strewn terrain, arms and hands close to the body, and a single pole occasionally making contact with the terrain at a variety of random points. This may explain comments I've received like, "I don't know what you're doing," "It doesn't look like you use the pole much."

Your STP allows you to efficiently keep your body erect and centered over each transition from the lead foot to the trailing foot while hiking, with minimal upper body and arm motion. It is literally as though you are "walking in the park."

Climbing with your STP improves efficiency by allowing the lead foot and leg only to lift your body. (**Figure 3-1**)

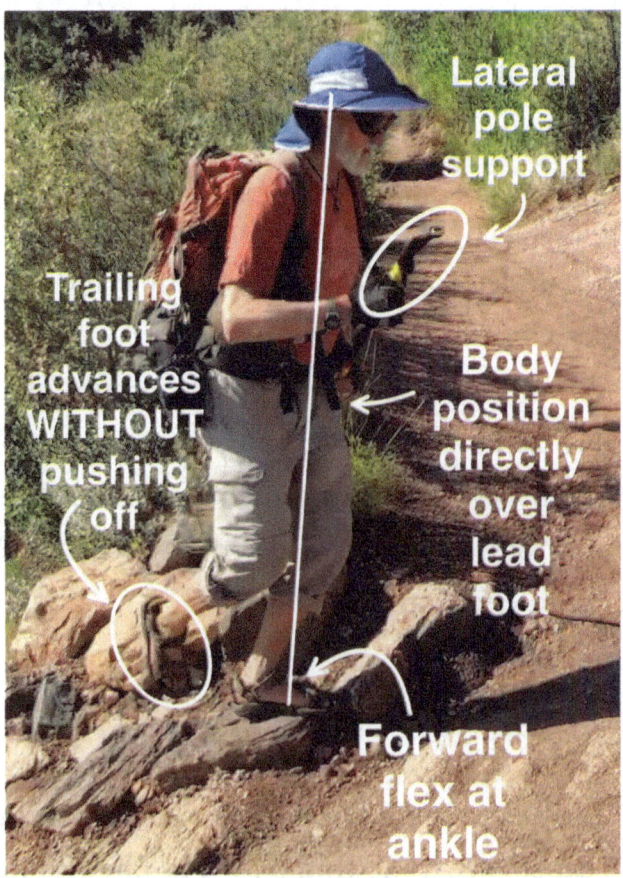

Fig. 3-1

Foot Placement and the Single Tall Pole

Your trailing foot should not lift for four reasons:

1) Your large thigh muscles are more than capable of lifting the body when your body is centered over the lead foot.

2) Lifting your body with your leading leg gives your trailing foot and leg a rest as you bring them forward.

3) Your trailing foot is immediately available to advance as soon as it is freed from supporting your weight on its full-foot position (i.e., heel down). Ideally, visualize: "When your lead foot engages, the trailing foot simultaneously disengages."

4) Lifting your body with the rear foot transfers weight forward on that foot, beyond most of the natural padding under the ball of your foot.

The ball of the foot is a joint. (**Figure 3-2**) Continually supporting your weight on this joint, particularly during long hikes or multi-day hikes, will eventually cause soreness if not damage to your feet.

I experienced unexplained soreness in my calves and balls of my feet backpacking three weeks on the John Muir Trail. After climbing numerous passes, I finally diagnosed and solved the problem. I was subconsciously lifting my body and pack weight using my trailing foot, all the while assuming my problem was caused by improper lead foot placements on descents. (Much later, I realized my subconscious tendency to lift my body onto the toes of my

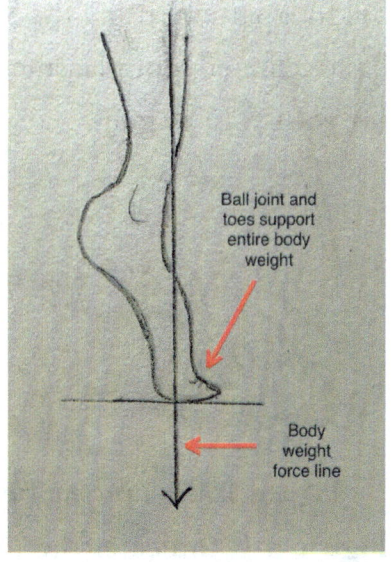

Fig. 3-2

lead foot as I advanced my trailing foot when I climbed stairs. It's a habit one can easily break. When climbing stairs, use the muscles of the leading leg to lift your body, keeping your heel down, while advancing your trailing leg to the next step above your leading leg. Raising your body onto the toes of your feet is extra work and will increase the stress on your toes.)

When climbing and hiking, try this mnemonic to advance your trailing foot: "Lead with the knee." This helps you quickly lift and advance your trailing foot, and prevents you from lifting your body with your toes. It also helps you simultaneously advance your hip and body so both are over your new lead foot when it contacts the ground.

Your ankles are continuously flexing to adjust to uneven hiking terrain. Through all of this, you maintain core bodyweight over each full foot pattern, using the Single Tall Pole. These three figures show basic centered foot placements that **maximize the terrain available for your foot to grip.**

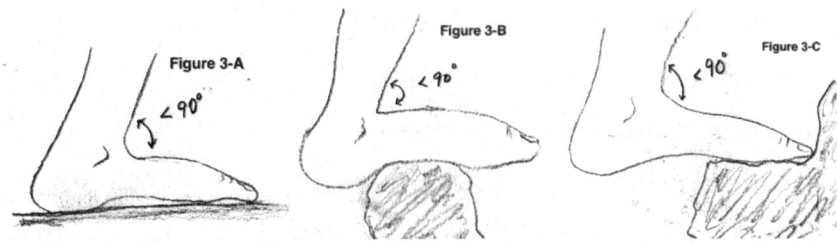

Figure 3-A is a proper position for both ascending or descending. **Figure 3-B** indicates the importance of centering your foot over variously shaped obstacles. **Figure 3-C** shows the importance of this foot position in allowing leg muscles to do the lifting AND **avoiding** rolling the body weight up onto the foot's ball joint. Note the forward flex at your ankles occurs because you are maintaining your athletic position over each foot placement, regardless of the difficulty of your climbing terrain. Your STP maintains your stability over each foot placement, giving you a bit of extra time to comfortably consider your next tip and foot placements. You shouldn't feel rushed or hurried in rugged terrain using your STP.

Observe two basic tip placements with respect to the pole's relationship to the hiker's body in the two **Figures 3-3** and **3-4**. The **lateral-forward** placement will have his guide hand out in front of his body, and his pressure hand will be near his chest. The **lateral-back** position will be the opposite, his guide hand near his hip with his pressure hand out behind and away from his body.

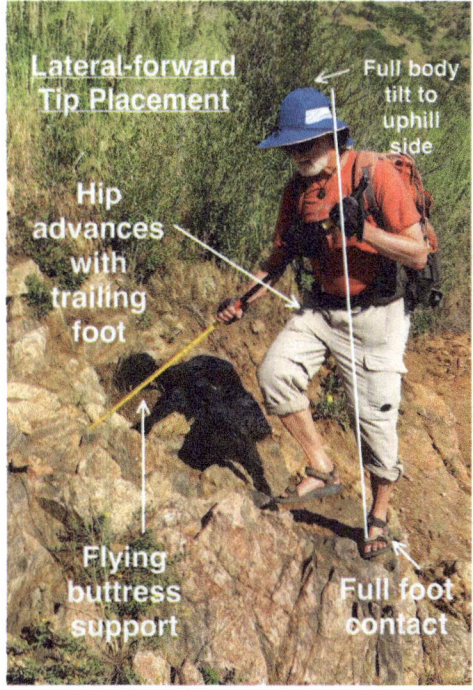

Fig. 3-3

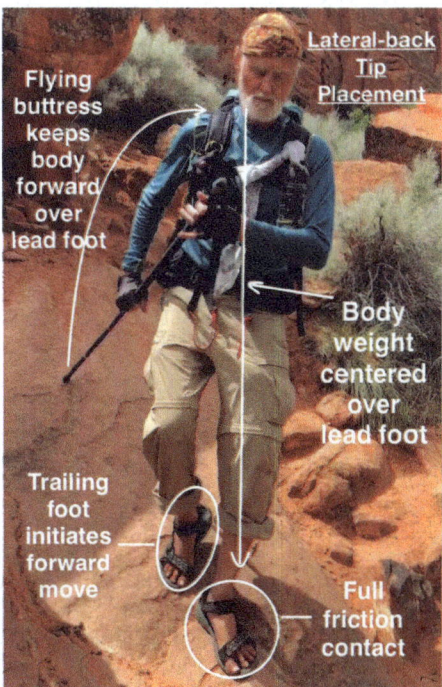

Fig. 3-4

Multiple variations within this fore and aft range lets him ascend and descend maintaining his bodyweight directly over each lead foot. The **lateral-forward** placement prevents him from leaning too far forward and stooping at the waist. The **lateral-back** tip placement counteracts his tendency to shift his bodyweight onto his heels.

You can make use of any of the wide range of variations between these two examples to quickly adjust, and exert just enough pressure on your STP to keep your body upright and centered in the athletic position over your lead foot.

When you are descending and staring down a steep slope, **it is imperative to keep your weight directly over your lead foot by slightly tilting your entire body forward with your hips — not hinging at the waist. This requires you to concentrate on slightly lowering your body to maintain forward flex in your ankles and knees.** If you are new to scrambling and friction climbing, this may seem and "feel" counterintuitive as you practice this technique.

Intermittent tapping of your STP tip behind you will occur each time the tendency to lean back occurs, signaling **"Hey you — stay focused!"** on the terrain directly under foot, and **not** on the deep river gorge below. If your mind wanders away from the feet, your weight may shift back onto your heels, and the tendency to initiate a swimmer's backstroke kicks in!

The following **Figures 3-5**, **3-6**, **3-7**, and **3-8** (on next page) illustrate the STP's "flying buttress" concept, using the basic STP techniques (Chapter 2) on a **high-step maneuver**. Note the hiker's body is upright and tilted toward the uphill-side of the terrain, reassuring the hiker he is solidly on the ground and won't fall in steep difficult terrain. This keeps the body weight centered over full-foot placements maximizing friction with the climbing surface.

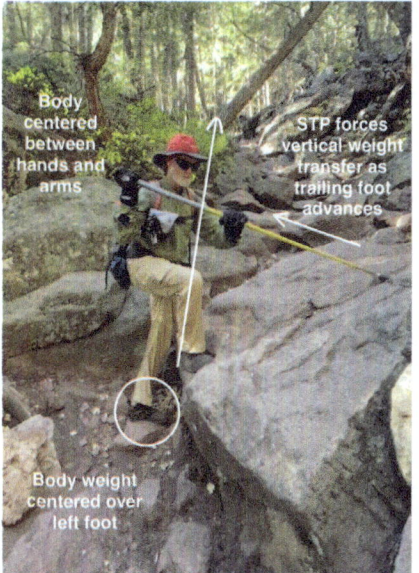

Fig. 3-5

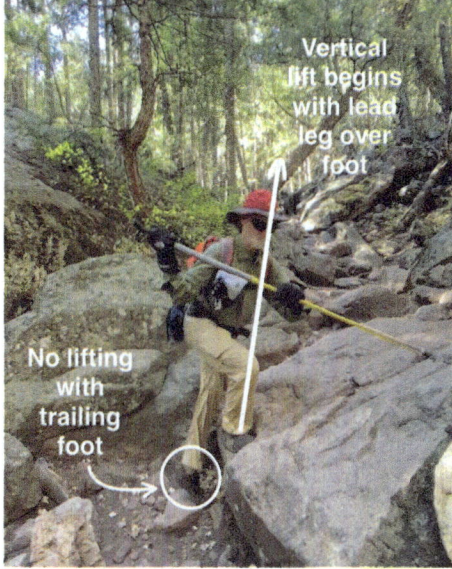

Fig. 3-6

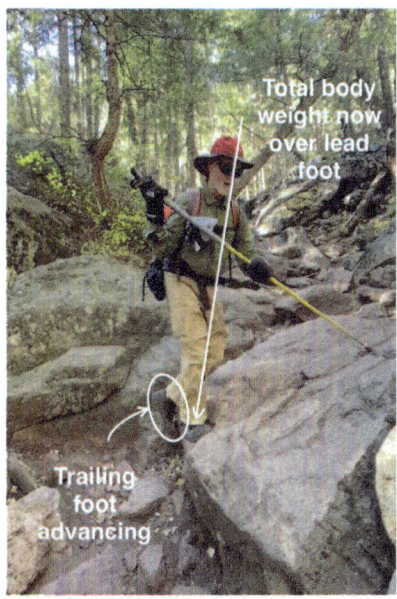

Fig. 3-7

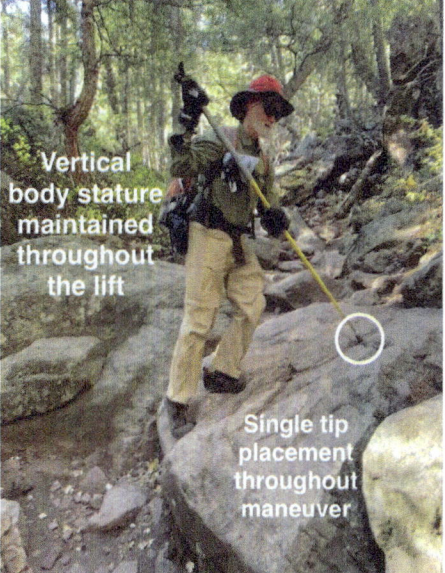

Fig. 3-8

Both hands firmly grip the STP to maintain force on your "flying buttress." This allows your larger leg muscles to lift your body upward, high enough to advance your trailing foot to the next lead-foot position. The "buttress" force back toward you blocks your tendency to hinge at the waist, which would change your core balance point and the amount of friction under your supporting foot. Also note, only one strategic tip placement is used throughout this maneuver.

There is a problem with strides that can occur in both ascending and descending, which I will refer to as "the reach." This can occur with either the lead or trailing foot. The reach is a common technique a climber uses when relying on two short hiking poles to support the body's center of gravity either fore or aft of a centered stable position over a full-foot placement.

On a descent, using a heel strike is by nature an impulsive braking action when you are staring down a steep slope. Your trailing leg's heel anchors your body while your lead foot "reaches" for placement. This means your lead foot and leg are ahead of your body's center of mass, making it impossible to keep your body upright and its weight over the forefoot of your lead foot, which significantly reduces your boot's grip on the terrain underneath. **(Figure 3-9)**

When the forefoot of your lead foot touches the ground, your body's forward momentum force is at a low angle to the terrain under foot. With your lead foot on a bit of loose sand or gravel it may slip, resulting in your fall. Also, in this case, both of your

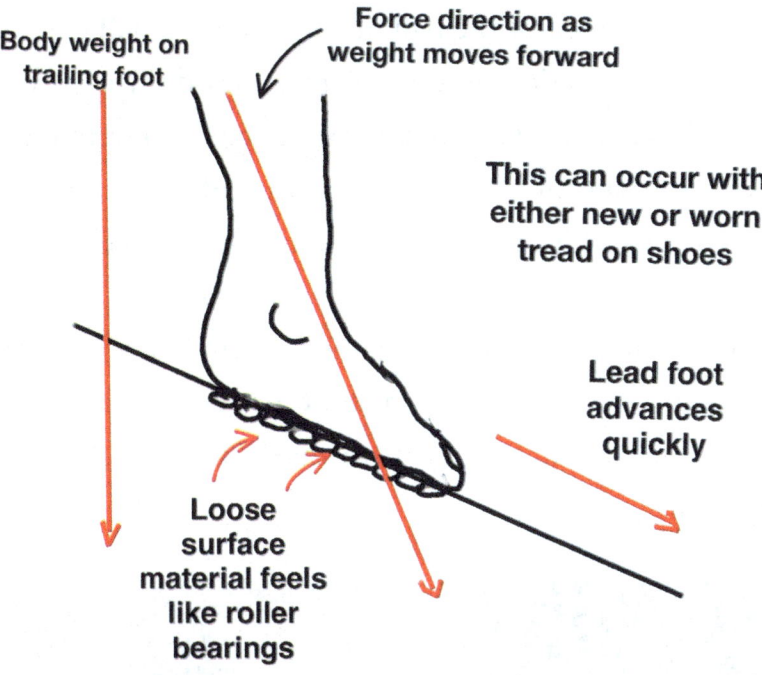

Fig. 3-9

foot placements may be precarious because your lead foot lacks perpendicular pressure for a sufficient friction hold, and your back foot heel may be anchoring the body's weight. You have doubled your chance for a fall, because you are relying for support on the minimal amount of contact the heel of your boot has with the ground.

On an ascent, the "reach" occurs on the trailing foot. In an effort to lengthen a stride, you may extend, or "reach," with your trailing leg by lifting your body up onto the ball joint of your trailing foot and toes. (**Figure 3-10**) Your weight has shifted forward, eliminating perpendicular pressure on your foot and minimizing your boot's grip on the ground.

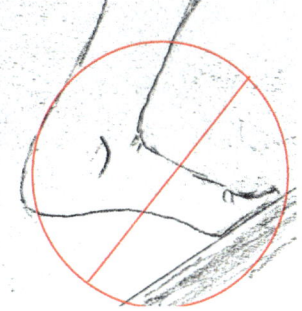

Fig. 3-10

The force on that foot is back down the slope at a low angle. Your boot's sole area in front of the ball of your foot is small enough, it may lack sufficient traction to support this forward thrust. Frequent trailing foot slips are inevitable in these situations — not to mention your frustrations and the useless expenditure of your energy.

You can prevent this by consciously keeping your heel in contact with the ground by using shorter steps, creative foot placements (**Figures 3-11** and **3-12**), and traveling low angle traverses across fall lines. Your direction change may be needed for only two or three strides, just enough for you to maximize your boot's grip on the ground.

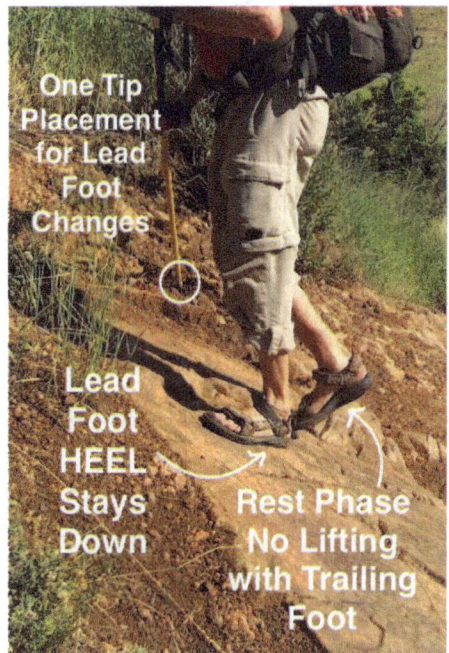

Fig. 3-11

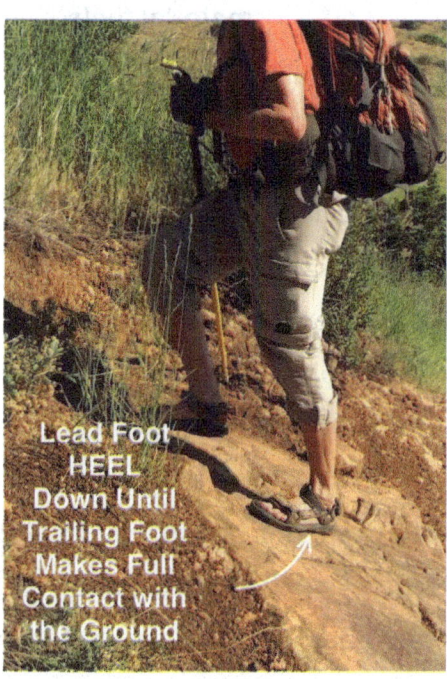

Fig. 3-12

You must continually adjust your technique for the terrain directly under foot. Climbers and hikers descending on loose, gravelly routes are wisely worried about loose debris causing a fall. You can learn to mitigate this worry.

Perform your own quick test on a very low angle, downward-sloping trail covered with gravel debris. This type of surface appears unstable for footing, which it can be. Stop, then place your lead foot with your full bodyweight, on it and a forward flex at the ankle onto the gravelly surface. You should feel your erect upper body is tilted slightly downhill. Notice there is little, if any, shifting under your foot.

Now try to make your foot shift while keeping your bodyweight directly over it. Also notice that the individual pieces of gravel are very angular in shape and not at like ball bearings — not even close. The friction grip is stable as long as your weight remains directly over your foot, causing those angular pieces to bite into the terrain.

While in this position, slowly shift your weight back to your trailing foot and notice how quickly your lead foot starts moving forward, and the stable gravel under your lead foot suddenly **feels like roller bearings**. "Oh my god, they changed shape on me!" (There's no "shapeshifting" in the backcountry!)

The feeling of roller bearings happens because your lead foot is not supporting your full bodyweight and therefore no longer forcing the angular gravel pieces to bite into the surface of the terrain. They are now easily moving under your foot. In fact, with light pressure from your hand, you could brush them aside. Maximum pressure begets maximum traction.

Use your STP while doing these simple foot placement tests on variable surfaces so you experience the "flying buttress" effect in maintaining a solid, stable feeling over each lead-foot exchange. Concentrate on your athletic stance, with a forward flex at the ankle, while testing to maximize friction underfoot. Your testing will give you confidence in the grip of your boots on all types of sloped surfaces.

The STP enables you to be creative with your foot placements, maximize traction, and avoid climbing on the balls of your feet. You can use these two step patterns examples for quick footing adjustment — the Cross-over step and the T-step.

Your **Cross-over step** starts with each foot at a comfortable upward angle across the fall line to maintain your full foot contact with the terrain. (**Figure 3-13**) You then place your downhill foot in front of the uphill foot to make a cross-over step pattern. You will gain elevation by bringing your trailing foot forward and placing it above and ahead of your downhill foot (i.e., lead foot) on each stride. Use a lateral-forward STP tip placement to maintain your core bodyweight over each lead foot placement. Your pole tip placements can be used for one or more strides across steep slopes.

Your STP tip placements also allow you to use the quick and easy **T-step pattern** (**Figure 3-14**) to maintain full foot contact on steep variable sections. Pressure on your STP keeps your knee and

Crossover Step

Ascend steep fall line maximizing full foot placements. Avoids climbing on balls of feet.

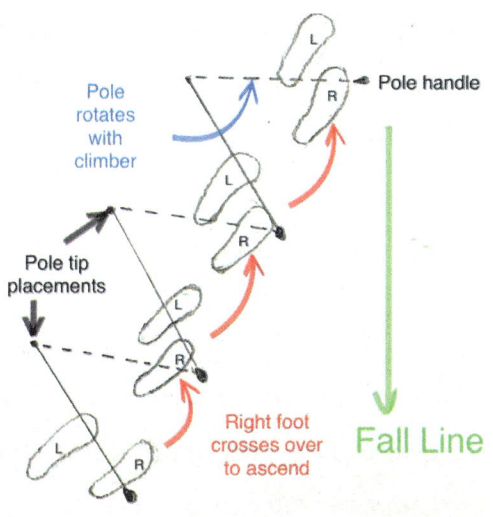

Fig. 3-13

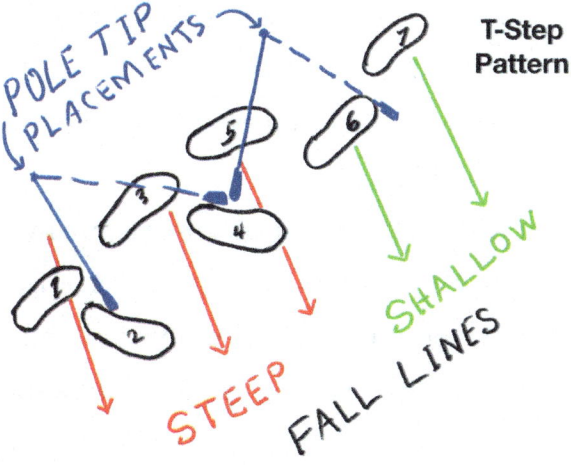

Fig. 3-14

ankle flexed over each lead foot exchange. In the figure, T-Steps #2 and #4 anchor steps #1, #3 and #5 as they advance. Your anchor feet maximize your boot's grip on the ground (with forward flex in your ankle) by rotating your leg at your hip and ankles in the direction of the fall line, thus allowing the lead foot placements to advance you across a slope. You can use variations of these foot patterns for either ascending or descending.

Traversing (ascending or descending) across a slope naturally requires side-to-side ankle flexion to help you maintain full foot contacts with the terrain. Flexible footwear encourages this.

Stiff-soled shoes or boots tend to cause hikers (like skiers) to use the edge of their boots rather than full foot placements to maintain traction, resulting in lots of slipping and trail damage in steep areas. Hikers also tend to orient their shoulders perpendicular to the fall line when using short double hiking poles, causing them to travel too steeply down the fall lines.

This is how steep "social trails" (non-professionally constructed trails) are created. They are sections of trails covered by all kinds of loosened rock and gravel, scraped and scoured by hikers slipping and sliding across these steep areas. It's where double-pole users are typically hinging at the waist, suspending their bodies out over their hiking poles, using their heels or the balls of their feet, poling with both arms to muscle their way through the steep terrain, expending unnecessary energy, straining to prevent falling because they are continually losing traction under their feet, not to mention possibly causing foot soreness within their boots. "Whew!"

You can comfortably circumvent many frustrating, steep "social trails" that send many hikers straight up or down fall lines on loose gravely terrain. Assuming the terrain is open enough, you can hike a short distance away from the trail using low-angle switchbacks. Lateral use of your STP makes your creative foot placements easier and allows you to make the length of your strides comfortable enough to keep your boot fully in contact with the ground. You minimize terrain damage by using full-foot contacts on your climbs. Additionally, your STP keeps you in a stable, upright position, expanding your view, and giving you more options to pick your way through gnarly terrain.

The best way to build your confidence using your STP is to practice on any trail or route. On easy trails there are numerous rocks sticking up all along the trails. You can take advantage of these rocks. Notice by looking at how the soil around them shows how many people avoid them — but not you! You want to learn the feel of your feet connecting with those rocks, the feel of stability you have using your STP to keep your body directly over your feet on those rocks. Make it a game for yourself, continually traveling across all the rock formations along your way. You will become well prepared to comfortably climb in more rugged terrain.

Generally speaking, you will use the lateral-forward pole position most often. By placing the tip of your STP in front of you, it continually provides you with support until you pass it, or it needs to be changed.

Practice tip placements more often than you think you need to. You are developing muscle memory, and learning how you feel over each foot on different shapes of rocks, roots, etc. Your proficiency will then allow you to concentrate on important immediate route finding, that is, over the next two to three feet for the next foot placements. The STP gives you time to make changes mid-stride, and your upright athletic position allows you to quickly evaluate your travel route even farther ahead.

The information presented in Chapters 2 and 3 provides a foundation on which we can expand those techniques to prevent numerous detrimental "plunge steps" that can occur on most hiking and climbing activities.

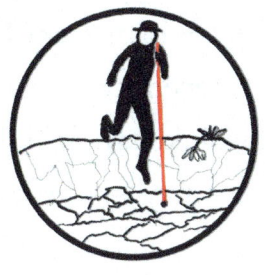

4

THE "PLUNGE STEP" AVOIDANCE

Everything should be made as simple as possible, but not simpler.
— Albert Einstein, physicist

I chose Einstein's quote because it illustrates the dynamics regarding the use of two short alpine ski poles for hiking and climbing.

Historically, climbers may have assumed their old alpine ski poles were a quick remedy to alleviate various symptoms of pain during their climbs. There may have been some benefit; however, over time, the use of these devices is now seen as a necessity for climbers, regardless of any pain they may experience. It is now a cultural meme within the outdoor crowd that, "You gotta use two hiking poles if you're going to climb or hike."

This meme lacks Einstein's logical process of using simple known techniques and a simple single device for more effective results. Einstein's term — "simpler" — applies to the use of short ski poles.

The short hiking poles are inefficient for hiking, and woefully ineffective at helping you prevent the detrimental effects of plunge stepping that occur on your hikes and climbs. You can easily ignore (particularly if you're in a hurry or getting tired) the continuous impacts on your joints of an inch or two and more of drop — especially when your full bodyweight, plus the additional weights of your daypacks and backpacks, drops (free falls) onto each lead foot during the numerous descents throughout your trips.

Larger drops occur on steeper, more difficult routes. Even on easier terrain, hikers with doubles poles may carry both in one hand or stash them on their packs, unaware of the cumulative effects small plunge steps have on their bodies.

Popping pain pills before, during, and after your hikes and backpacks shouldn't be your first line of defense. You can effectively use your STP to eliminate plunge stepping on any trail or climbing route.

Think of your STP as a preventive measure against joint pain, rather than waiting for pain to dictate a necessary change in your technique.

I learned many years ago on my first week-long backpack into the Grand Canyon (without using poles) just how quickly one can damage joints. This was before outdoor shops considered selling ski poles as hiking poles. I plunge stepped down a steep trail with big steps designed for mules. The descent seemed easy enough, but I was traveling too fast with a very heavy backpack.

After a rest break at less than five miles, both knees suddenly seemed to flame in extreme pain. I hobbled the next five miles or so on the relatively level Tonto Trail before needing a layover day to recuperate enough to continue. My thoughts were: "Can I even get out of the canyon?" "Will this be my last backpack?"

Before my trip, I read Colin Fletcher's book, ***The Man Who Walked Through Time,*** about his experiences as the first person to walk the length of the Grand Canyon. He wrote of the importance of using a single tall pole.

To my peril, I ignored his advice.

We crossed paths with a few experienced Canyon backpackers who explained the necessity of using the single tall bamboo poles which they were using to prevent plunge stepping. Realizing how fast my damage occurred, my goal since has been to prevent plunge stepping on ANY trail or climbing route, REGARDLESS of the difficulty of the terrain. The STP has allowed me to adapt my climbing techniques and achieve my goals without experiencing any more impact than if I were descending a flight of stairs without a pack. I now have over 35 week-long backpacks into the Grand Canyon, in addition to many multiple day hikes there.

You need to control the way you transfer your bodyweight from the rear foot to the lead foot with minimal impact to prevent the detrimental plunge step. You will see how the techniques discussed in the previous chapters need to be adjusted, because you are now trying to prevent your total bodyweight from free falling onto your lead foot each time you step down a big drop.

To start, evaluate your technique descending stairs. Your lead forefoot makes the initial contact with the step below as you descend.

That initial contact activates the muscles of your foot and leg to suspend and gently lower your body's weight onto a full footprint. You can easily transfer this technique to the backcountry because you have been using it for years.

People don't tend to plunge step down stairs, unless their ages are in the 10-12 year range. Many hikers tend to accept small and large plunge steps as just a part of hiking. Your short hiking poles are not conducive to dealing with plunge steps unless you disregard what we've covered so far in this book.

If you want to prevent unnecessary potential injury while climbing and hiking, for your long-term benefit, learning to use your STP is a very helpful tool.

You may alternate between two different STP tip placement methods to prevent plunge steps when you are descending trails or off-trail routes with varying step heights in close succession. (**Figure 4-1**)

1. You may use lateral STP tip placements (lateral-back and lateral-forward, Chapter 3) to prevent short descent plunge steps (less than a foot) by **slightly changing your position** when you initiate this move. You place the STP tip so you are able to keep your bodyweight over your back foot. Your **back leg muscles** slow your descent just long enough to allow the forefoot of your lead foot to touch the ground, activating the muscles in your foot and leg and gently transferring your bodyweight onto your entire foot.

The "Plunge Step" Avoidance

You do so without breaking your stride and rhythm hiking along the trail.

2. To avoid plunge steps off steep steps or drop-offs (about one half to two feet), you need to add a special, simple STP technique to your repertoire — the **single (hand-arm-shoulder) support unit.**

Your STP's extra length gives you the advantage of engaging your upper body core muscles, using one arm to place the pole tip — a single arm tip placement — to prevent a plunge step. Your initial strategic tip placement allows you to start the maneuver with a right-angle bend at your arm's elbow while maintaining your upright body position. You are now set

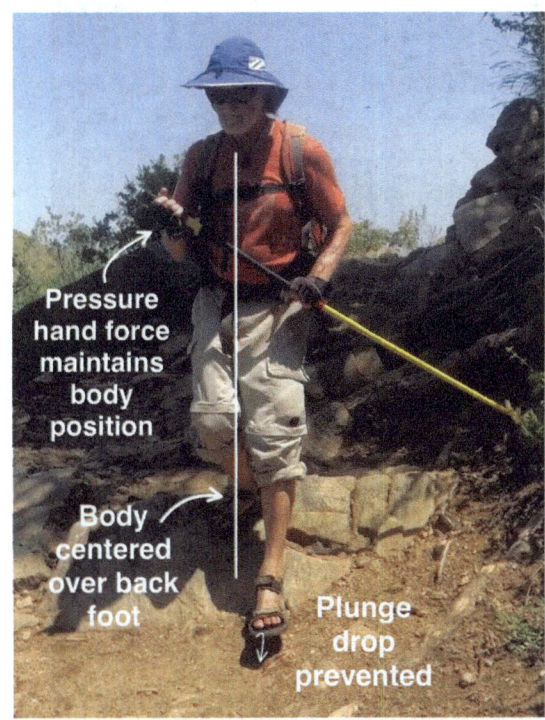

Fig. 4-1

up to maintain your upright posture through the descent. This method enables you to quickly adjust the position of your grip on your STP to any descending step distance.

Let me walk you through the process. (**Figures 4-2** and **4-3**, on the next page) Your pole is held vertically in front of you, with one hand near its midsection. There is neither a guide hand nor pressure

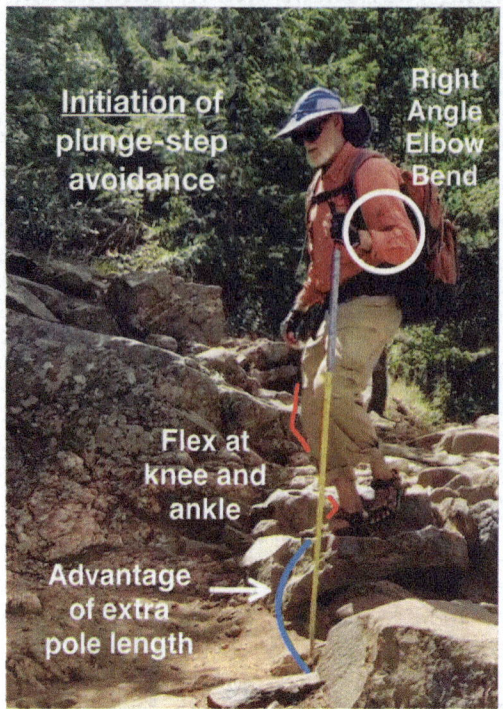

Fig. 4-2

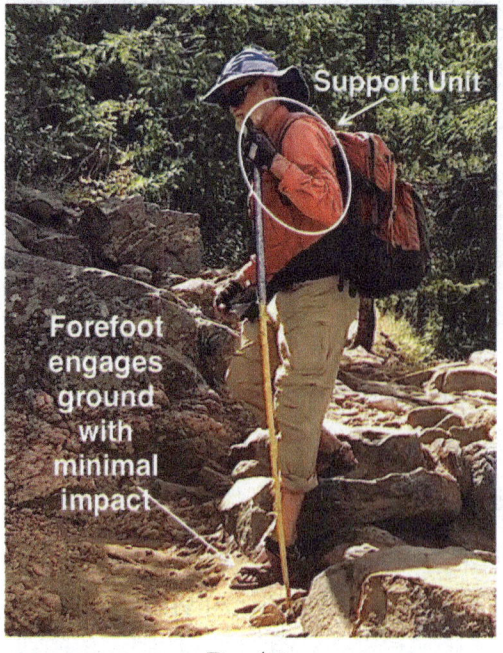

Fig. 4-3

hand in this maneuver. At the top of a drop-off or big step, you relax your grip to allow your STP to quickly slip through your fingers to engage the tip at the bottom of the step. You then grasp your pole at or near the top handle to strategically place its tip near the front area of your travel. As your lead foot advances to descend, your bodyweight is briefly supported over your back foot. As you start descending, your hand grips the pole and your arm muscles tighten, drawing your STP's handle close to your shoulder and chest. Your "single arm (hand-arm-shoulder) support unit," in combination with your back leg, effectively uses your STP to briefly suspend and lower your body until the lead forefoot engages the ground below. **You effectively change a plunge step to a**

simple transfer of your bodyweight from one well-grounded foot on a higher level to another well grounded foot on a lower level as though you are traveling on level ground. You maintain an efficient, upright, athletic position throughout the process, and eliminate impact on your feet, knees, and back.

If a larger descent step is required, you allow the terrain to determine which hand to use and where you place the pole tip forward of your position. Many times your single-arm tip placement may be made at or near the bottom of the large drop or step, allowing you to create a single arm support unit to take several smaller steps down into the large step. You may slide your hand downward as needed along your STP as you progress until reaching the bottom. Your hand change will become intuitive with experience as you maneuver through your strides without delay.

Your properly-sized STP's extra length approximates the maximum distance your leg can reach below on a steep step or drop-off using your single-arm support unit. It's to your advantage to make an oversized STP rather than accepting anything less than your properly sized measure.

You may use a more relaxed version of the single-arm support unit on shorter steps or lower angle descents to easily maintain your maximum traction under each foot. Note the hiker's right-angle bend at his elbow in the initiation (**Figure 4-4,** on the next page) and the shift to a lower hand grip position (**Figure 4-5,** on the next page) during the steps of his descent, all using the same STP tip placement. Also note, his relaxed upright body stature is maintained through the descent. You may shift your hand position on your STP anytime you are centered over secure foot placements

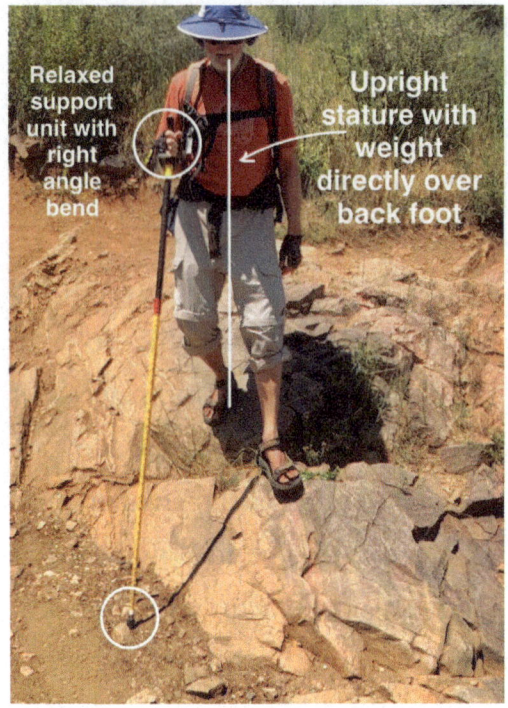

Fig. 4-4

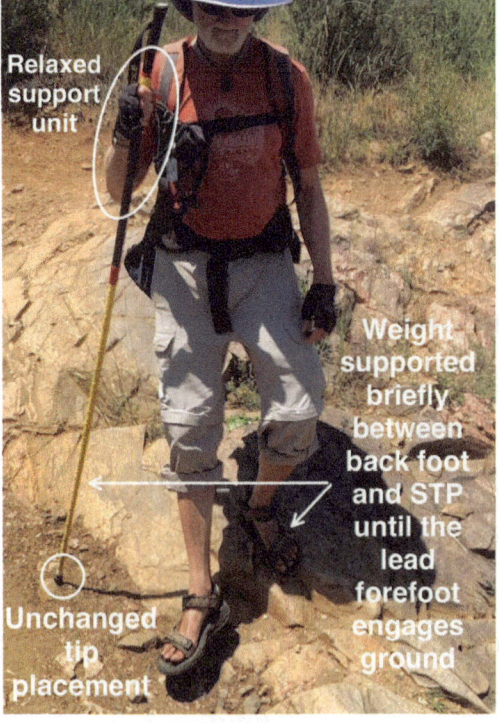

Fig. 4-5

during stride transitions. This flexibility allows you to have the proper pole length at all times to meet your ever changing needs.

You can avoid continuously plunge stepping on sections of trail with boulders or multiple water bars. As you approach each step, you decide which poling hand is needed for the best tip and foot placements. Then, with that hand, let the STP slide through your fingers to set its tip on the step below. (The wrist strap acts as a stop preventing dropping your pole during quick tip placement maneuvers.) Grasp your STP, engage your single-arm support unit and your back leg muscles, and lower your body onto the forefoot of your leading foot. Once you are fully supported on your lead foot, relax your grip on the STP and slide your hand down to its midpoint so you are holding it in a vertical neutral position. You now have time to decide if you want to use the same hand to set the tip of your STP for the next step, or switch it to your other hand. With practice, the best tip and foot placements will become obvious, and you will be able to decide quickly which hand to use to set the tip of your STP.

You can test this process by using your STP going down a set of stairs. Let the STP quickly slide through your fingers to set the tip two steps below you each time you descend a single step. Using your single-arm support unit and the large leg muscles of your back leg, lower your front foot onto the next step below. You may use the same hand, or occasionally switch hands, all the way to the bottom of the stairs.

This technique for descending steep steps on the trail accomplishes three things: 1) It allows you to make quick tip placements, 2) It gives your large leg and torso muscles control of your descent down each step, 3) It eliminates the detrimental effects of plunge stepping on your body by converting a steep chain of drops into a descent which feels like a comfortable walk on level terrain.

Your STP is a tool. You will become creative at using it to keep your body upright in your athletic position, which makes it easier for you to place your feet in the most solid, stable positions on your climbs and hikes. You will become very aware of the amount of unnecessary stress, strain, and impact you previously accepted as "just part of the outdoor experience."

NOTE TO BACKPACKERS

Some backpackers incorporate their hiking poles into their tent structures in place of their tent poles in an effort to shave a few ounces off their pack weights. This is a non-issue when hiking with your STP. Your STP is always available for a side hike or climb after your tent is set and ready for inclement weather. Your personal hiking efficiency, increased energy and decreased fatigue at the end of the day is paramount to reducing your pack weight by the few ounces tent poles weigh, especially on long distance trips.

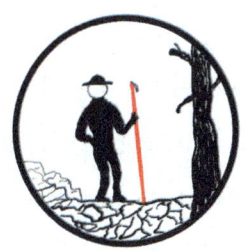

5
ADAPTING A SKI POLE

SUPPLIES AND EQUIPMENT

POLE PREPARATION
Ski pole
Rubber cane tip
Duct tape and hot glue stick
Hacksaw and hot water
Utility knife

HANDLE PREPARATION
Double stick Scotch Tape (or similar strong double stick tape)
Bicycle handlebar tape/wrap (inexpensive, road racing-style)
Electrical tape

An Internet search for tall poles resulted in finding dual purpose poles, monopod-trekking pole combinations. These are predominantly used for photography, spotting scopes, or rifle supports. Some list maximum support weights of about ten to 13 pounds. They are light weight, adjustable, and designed to be used for trekking, similar to standard short hiking poles. Even if the monopods extend to your proper height measurement, they may not be designed to support your bodyweight pressure applied to your STP during climbs or plunge step avoidance maneuvers.

The choice of a tall ski pole is important. It is designed to support a skier's full bodyweight pressure onto the poles under ski racing conditions.

Your STP must be sized properly for you to attain the maximum benefits from its use. **Your STP's extra length, beyond the traditional short hiking poles' lengths, approximates the maximum useful downward distance your extended leg must reach to your lower foot placement position, using your single-arm support unit to prevent the plunge step. (Chapter 4)**

You may be tempted to try an undersized STP to see if you really want to fully commit to the STP method. Your test results will be inadequate and may cause you to give up on using a single tall pole. It's not too dissimilar from putting one of your hiking poles on your daypack and using only one slightly longer pole.

Your properly-sized STP greatly increases the range available for choosing your tip placements, which maintains your athletic position, which in turn maximizes your bodyweight directly over your feet, thus maximizing (the all important!) traction under your feet. **Maximizing your climbing efficiency is predicated on using an STP of proper length.**

Your converted cross-country ski pole becomes a lightweight maneuverable tool. This allows you to quickly maneuver your STP'S tip to the proper placement position with single wrist actions of your guide hand (Chapter 2). You should reject any pole that has an alpine ski handle and adjustment devices like clips or clamps, as all will interfere with your ability to make quick, smooth hand position changes.

Ski poles come in pairs, so you will have a backup on hand. Do not remove your wrist strap from the cross-country ski pole, as you will find it very useful (Chapters 2 and 4).

The ski pole should be sized at about 90 percent of your height, approximately between your mouth and forehead. You will remove your ski pole's sharp point, which may make it shorter, so choose a longer length if you're selecting between two close sizes.

A top-of-the-line ski racing pole is not necessary. Basic new ski pole models or second-hand ski poles are available at many ski and outdoor shops. Many new ski poles, fiberglass and aluminum, are relatively inexpensive. (An Internet search reveals ski skating poles up to 175cm/69in. in length.)

Rubber cane tips (5/8 inch) are readily available on the Internet, some pharmacies, and medical supply shops. The rubber cane tips are designed to provide friction support and safety for users with special medical needs. Avoid chair and table leg tips, which may be designed to slide effortlessly across floors. You are looking for friction support.

The shafts of most ski poles are 5/8 inch in diameter or less. Five different variations of ski tips are shown in the picture. (**Figure 5-1**)

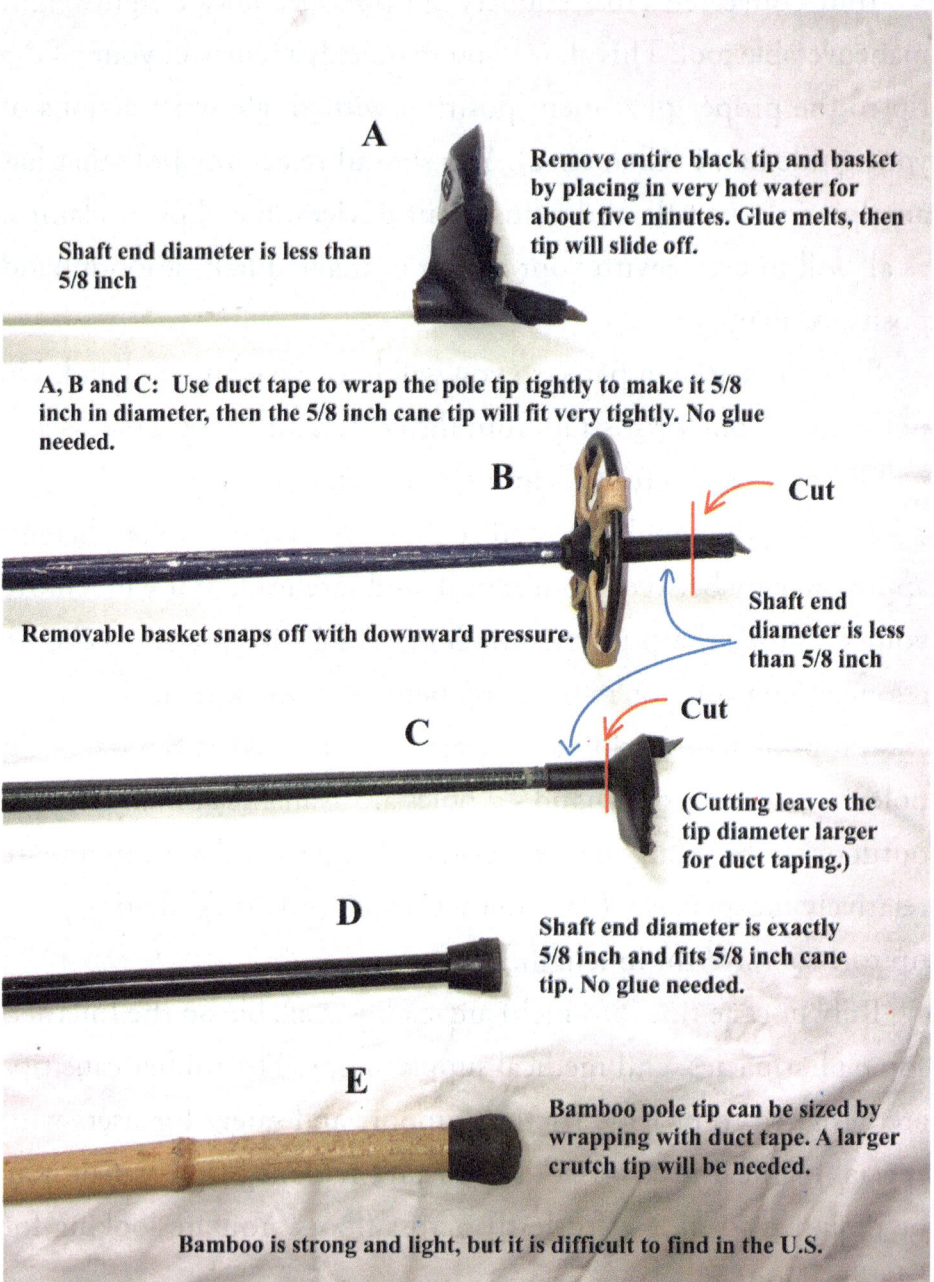

Fig. 5-1

Tip A can be removed by placing it in a small pot of very hot water (not boiling) for about three to five minutes. The glue softens, and the entire unit can be pulled off. Leave it in the hot water a little longer if it still seems hard to remove. Any residual glue on the shaft is a non-issue. (To my surprise, I did find a ski pole similar to "Tip A" that was permanently glued and would not come off with the hot water treatment. I had to saw the tip and basket off with a hacksaw.)

Tips B and C may be cut off with a hacksaw to preserve a larger diameter on the shaft near the tip end. The basket on Tip B snaps into a grove, so with a bit of pressure it will pop off.

Shaft D's tip was removed using hot water. The shaft is the same size as the rubber tip (5/8 inch), which can be forced on the shaft immediately. If the rubber tip doesn't fit tightly (i.e., very tightly), and there's not enough room to use duct tape, use the hot glue stick glue on the shaft end and quickly force the rubber tip on before it cools.

Tips A, B and C have diameters less than 5/8 inch. The diameter of the shaft can be increased by a few tight wraps of duct tape to create a very tight fit for the cane tip without gluing. **Force the rubber tip onto the shaft end to its full depth.** Make it fit very tightly. Any duct tape above the top of the rubber tip can be trimmed off with a utility cutter or knife.

I have not had any problem with the duct tape and rubber tip falling off during use even after multiple mud and stream crossings. In fact, when the rubber tip wears out, I have to cut off the rubber tip and duct tape with a utility knife, and then re-wrap the pole tip portion for the new rubber tip.

Sometimes the cut-off ends of some poles may not be perfectly round. In lieu of duct tape, which might make a portion of the pole end too large and the final end point too narrow, use the heat gun glue stick on the narrower sides to fill the space around it so there is total glue contact with the pole and the inside of the cane tip. This is the same glue that holds the spike tips on ski poles, which can be removed with the hot water bath mentioned above.

The last step is wrapping the upper 40-50 percent of the STP with bicycle handlebar tape. This provides a smooth grip area that allows quick hand transitions along the pole. You will need a roll of double-stick Scotch Tape. Buy bicycle handlebar tape designed to cover the curved handlebars of a road racing-style bike. (Tape for straight bike handlebars will be too short.) Any inexpensive handlebar tape will work. There will be a pair in the package, but only one is needed for your STP. Save the other one as a backup.

The first step is to **test wrap** your STP with the bike handlebar tape from the bottom of the fixed ski handle **downward** and mark where the wrap ends with a piece of duct tape (**Figure 5-2**). This will be the starting point for the final **upward** wrap to the ski handle. Both the test wrapping and final wrapping should be done by overlapping the tape by 1/3 on each round around the pole. The final upward wrapping creates a shingle-like layering of bike tape that will help it withstand downward hand pressure on the pole. You may need to do a couple of test wraps to get the end point marked correctly.

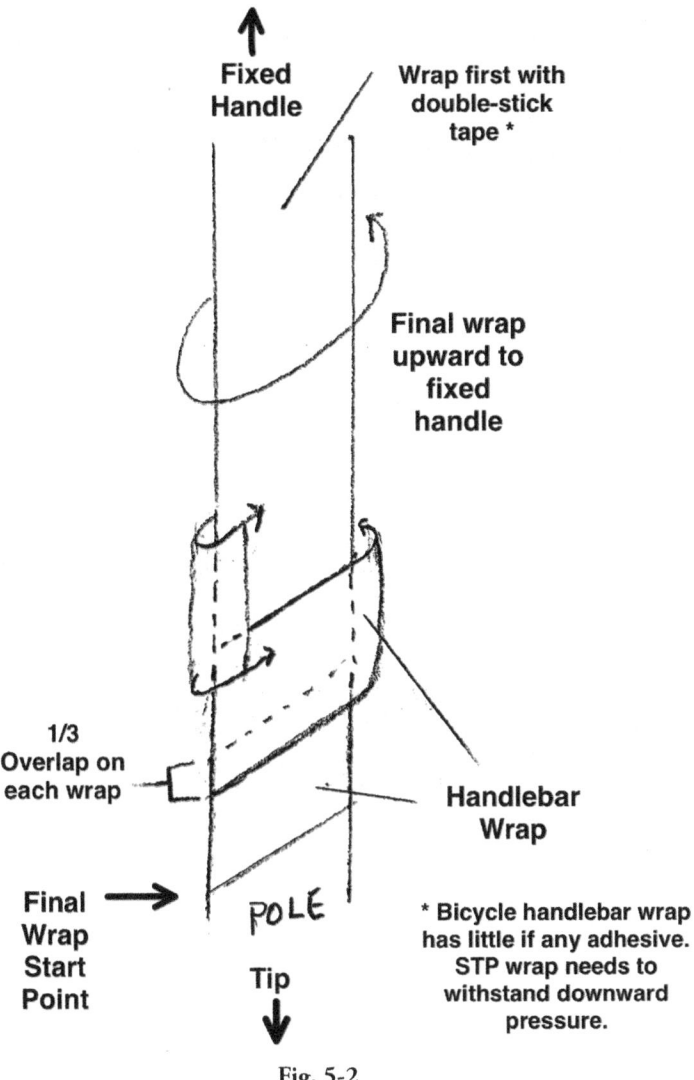

Fig. 5-2

Now use the double-stick Scotch Tape to circularly wrap the entire area from the bottom edge of the fixed handle down to your test wrap end point. You don't need to overlap the Scotch Tape or worry about wrinkles as your wrapping progresses. This can be taped in either direction. Bicycle handlebar tape has either no adhesive, or a weak adhesive, because cyclists' hands aren't putting significant pressure horizontally across their handlebars. The bike tape provides a solid padded grip area on the cyclist's steel handlebar, which also works very well for your STP.

The final wrap begins at your lower handle duct tape mark. Anchor the handlebar tape here with a piece of duct tape. Then wrap **tightly upward** overlapping about 1/3 of the wrap on each rotation. Take time wrapping; but if adjustment is needed, one can unwrap part way, if necessary, or even start over. Temporarily anchor this upper end with a piece of tape next to the fixed handle.

Finally, anchor each end of this segment tightly with several rotations of electrical tape. (Cut this tape with a knife. Do not tear with your fingers because stretching and finger prints will reduce the strength of the adhesive. Electrical tape, if not stretched, is very weather resistant and lasts.)

You now have an elegant Single Tall Pole.

EPILOGUE

I adapted willingly to the single tall pole after quickly developing two flaming knees due to plunge stepping on a backpack trip. (You don't need to try and break my record of inflaming both knees in under five miles!)

In my concerted effort to prevent plunge stepping on any subsequent trips, I soon realized how effective the STP was at providing stability over foot placements, beyond just plunge steps. It allowed me to be more efficient in reading the terrain immediately around my feet and farther ahead, to micro adjust climbing routes on the way to my desired destination. It made me aware of all the unnecessary stress, strain, and impact on my body, which I no longer need to tolerate as "just the price of being a climber or hiker."

It takes personal initiative to start making a properly-sized STP, and then some patience evaluating your stability while you adapt to using it. Stability is something you feel, but is difficult for an observer to detect.

Test yourself across any rocky areas available on a route. I believe "rock is your friend." With proper foot placement, you are far more stable on rock than loose dirt, gravel, or sand.

Challenge yourself on off-trail routes by setting comfortable low angle ascents and descents on ridges and high points. You will experience how effectively the Single Tall Pole enables you to expand your athletic climbing and hiking skills, comfortably, across multiple terrain types, with your efficient athletic position.

Here's to Faster, Longer, More Efficient, and Safer Climbing and Hiking!

And — Cheers To Your New Adventure!

Blake

ABOUT THE AUTHOR

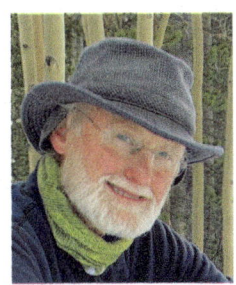

Stuart Blake Clark is a retired pharmacist and was a cofounding partner of Home I.V. Services, Inc. in 1982, which pioneered the concept of the administration of intravenous medications to patients in their homes following surgical hospitalizations. As a result, stabilized patients were able to avoid extended hospital stays in order to receive multiple weeks of required infusions.

Blake has been hiking with a Single Tall Pole (STP) since his initial backpack (c.a. 1990) into the Grand Canyon. He has since taken more than 35 week-long backpack trips there. He continues to use his STP on all hikes, on and off-trails, talus slopes, boulder fields, backpacks, and peak climbs (including on 3rd and 4th class routes and Colorado's 14,000-foot peaks). As a trip leader for the Colorado Mountain Club (CMC), he has been teaching backcountry cross country skiing for 25 years. For this, he took more than forty Professional Ski Instructors Association (PSIA) training clinics.

This book on the intricacies of using the Single Tall Pole for efficiency and greater safety is a culmination of Blake's experiences climbing, barefoot running, backpacks in the Grand Canyon, and teaching classic cross-country skiing — all of which he believes have a common thread.

Made in the USA
Coppell, TX
11 February 2026